IMPORTANT OF HEALTHY EATING HABITS FOR KIDS AND ADULTS

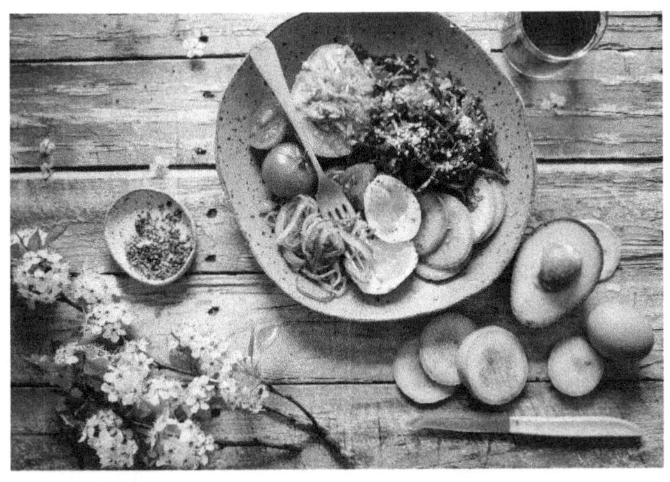

A Beginner's Guide To Nutritious Delicious Meal

Dr. Margaret M. Guido

TABLE OF CONTENT

Introduction

There lived a young boy named Alex who lived in a bustling little town of Nutriville. Alex was an energetic and curious child who loved exploring the world around him. However, he had a penchant for sugary treats, fast food, and skipping meals. Little did he know that his eating habits were affecting his overall well-being.One sunny day, while Alex was playing at the park, he noticed a peculiar-looking fruit stand. It was run by an elderly man called Mr. Greenleaf, who had a warm smile and a twinkle in his eyes. The colorful array of fruits and vegetables caught Alex's attention, and he approached the stand with curiosity."Hello, young lad!" Mr. Greenleaf greeted him cheerfully. "Can you try some fresh and nutritious fruits?"Alex's eyes widened as he examined the juicy apples, vibrant berries, and plump oranges. He couldn't resist and took a bite of a succulent strawberry. Instantly, a burst of flavor exploded in his mouth, and he felt invigorated.

Curiosity piqued, Alex started asking Mr. Greenleaf about the benefits of eating healthy foods. Mr. Greenleaf explained that healthy eating habits provide vital nutrients that fuel the body, enhance growth and development, and boost immunity. He emphasized that eating a balanced diet with plenty of fruits, vegetables, whole grains, and lean proteins would help Alex become stronger and more resilient.As days went by, Alex visited Mr. Greenleaf's fruit stand regularly, gradually replacing his sugary snacks with wholesome options. He discovered the joy of preparing meals with his parents using fresh ingredients. Together, they cooked colorful stir-fries, crunchy salads, and delicious smoothies. Alex realized that healthy eating was not only nourishing but also enjoyable.

With his newfound energy and improved focus, Alex excelled in school and sports. His friends and family noticed his positive transformation and began adopting healthier habits themselves. The once-lively town of Nutriville started embracing nutritious foods, and Mr. Greenleaf's fruit stand became the heart of the community.

Over time, Alex grew into a knowledgeable young man passionate about healthy living. He became an advocate for nutritious eating, organizing workshops and educating others on the importance of making smart food choices. Alex's journey from a boy with unhealthy eating habits to a beacon of health and vitality inspired those around him to lead healthier lives.From that day forward, the people of Nutriville embraced the significant impact of healthy eating habits. They understood that nourishing their bodies with wholesome foods not only made them feel good but also ensured a brighter future for themselves and their community.

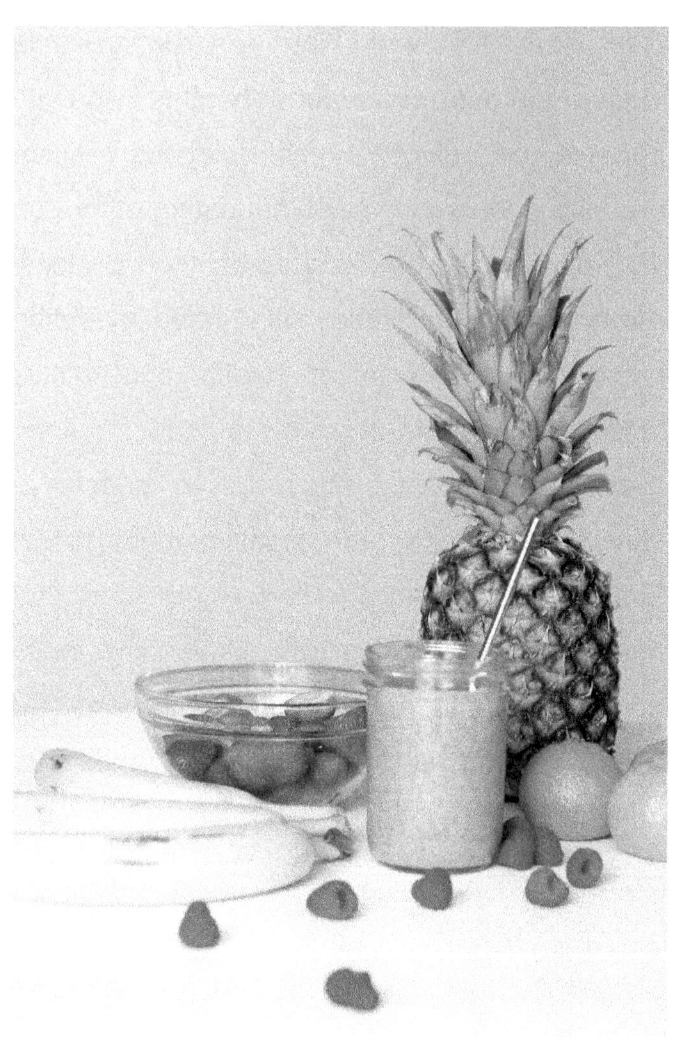

CHAPTER 1: HEALTHY EATING HABITS

Healthy eating habits refers to a set of practices and choices related to food that promote the overall well-being and support optimal physical and mental health. It involves consuming a balanced diet that includes a variety of nutrient-dense foods while maintaining appropriate portion sizes. Healthy eating habits emphasize the importance of incorporating fruits, vegetables, whole grains, lean proteins, and healthy fats into one's diet, while limiting the intake of processed foods, added sugars, unhealthy fats, and excessive salt. Also, healthy eating habits involve mindful eating, paying attention to hunger and fullness cues, staying adequately hydrated, and practicing moderation in food choices. By adopting and consistently following healthy eating habits, individuals can nourish their bodies, maintain a healthy weight, reduce the risk of chronic diseases, and enhance their overall quality of life.

Healthy eating habits play a crucial role in promoting the overall well-being. The following are some key reasons on why they are very important:

1.Nutritional Balance: Healthy eating habits ensure that your body receives a balanced intake of essential nutrients, including vitamins, minerals, proteins, carbohydrates, and fats. This helps support proper bodily functions, such as cell repair, immune system functioning, and energy production.

2.Disease Prevention: A well-balanced diet rich in fruits, vegetables, whole grains, and lean proteins can help reduce the risk of chronic diseases such as heart disease, diabetes, obesity, and certain types of cancer. It provides the necessary nutrients and antioxidants that support a healthy immune system and combat inflammation.

3.Weight Management: Healthy eating habits contribute to maintaining a healthy weight. By consuming nutrient-dense foods and controlling portion sizes, you can avoid excessive calorie intake and the associated weight gain. This, in turn, reduces the risk of obesity and its associated health complications.

4.Energy and Mental Well-being: Proper nutrition from healthy eating habits provides the energy required for daily activities and supports mental well-being. A balanced diet can help regulate blood sugar levels, improve focus and concentration, enhance mood stability, and reduce the risk of mental health conditions such as depression and anxiety.

5.Digestive Health: A diet rich in fiber, obtained from fruits, vegetables, and whole grains, promotes healthy digestion and prevents constipation. It also supports a diverse gut microbiome, which is linked to better immune function and improved overall health.

6.Longevity and Quality of Life: Adopting healthy eating habits can contribute to a longer and healthier life. By reducing the risk of chronic diseases, maintaining a healthy weight, and nourishing your body with essential nutrients, you enhance your overall quality of life and increase your chances of living a longer, more vibrant life

In summary, healthy eating habits plays a vital role for overall well-being as they provide the necessary nutrients, help prevent diseases, support weight management, enhance energy levels and mental health, improve digestion, and promote longevity.

The importance of a guide on healthy eating habits is to provide readers with valuable information, guidance, and practical tips to help them adopt and maintain a nutritious and balanced diet. Using the following guide:

1.Understanding the Fundamentals: The guide will explain the basic principles of healthy eating, including the importance of balanced nutrition, portion control, and the role of various food groups. It also provides clarity on macronutrients (carbohydrates, proteins, and fats) and micronutrients (vitamins and minerals) and their importance in maintaining overall health.

2.Nutrient-Rich Food Choices: The guide will highlight specific food items that are rich in essential nutrients, such as fruits, vegetables, whole grains, lean proteins, and healthy fats. It may include recommendations for portion sizes and suggestions for incorporating these foods into meals and snacks.

3.Meal Planning and Preparation: Readers can expect guidance on meal planning and preparation strategies, including tips for grocery shopping, meal prepping, and making healthier food choices when dining out. The guide may offer sample meal plans or recipe ideas to inspire nutritious and flavorful meals.

4.Mindful Eating Practices: The importance of mindful eating will likely be discussed, including techniques to promote conscious eating, such as paying attention to hunger and fullness cues, practicing portion control, and savoring each bite. Readers may also find advice on avoiding emotional or stress-related eating.

5.Addressing Dietary Restrictions or Preferences: The guide might touch upon various dietary patterns, such as vegetarianism, veganism, gluten-free diets, or specific allergen considerations. It may provide insights on meeting nutritional needs while adhering to these restrictions or preferences.

6.Long-Term Lifestyle Habits: A comprehensive guide will emphasize the importance of making healthy eating habits a long-term lifestyle choice rather than a short-term diet. It may address behavior change, goal setting, and practical tips for overcoming challenges or setbacks.

7.Supporting Overall Well-being: Readers can expect information on how healthy eating habits contribute to overall well-being, including benefits for physical health, mental health, energy levels, and disease prevention. The guide may also explore the connection between diet and other lifestyle factors such as exercise and sleep.

CHAPTER 2: UNDERSTANDING THE BASIC OF NUTRITION

MACRONUTRIENTS

Macronutrients are the essential nutrients required by the human body in large quantities to provide energy, support growth, and maintain overall health. The intake of macronutrients is essential for a well-rounded diet. The appropriate proportions of carbohydrates, proteins, and fats may vary depending on individual needs, goals, and dietary preferences. It's important to consider both the quality and quantity of macronutrients to maintain optimal health and support bodily functions.Macronutrients are the three major components of our diet that provide energy and are required in relatively large quantities. They include carbohydrates, proteins, and fats.

Carbohydrates:

Carbohydrates are the body's primary source of energy. They are found in foods such as grains (rice, bread, pasta), fruits, vegetables, legumes, and dairy products. We have two types of carbohydrates: simple and complex. Simple carbohydrates, like sugars, are quickly digested and provide rapid energy. Complex carbohydrates, like whole grains and starchy vegetables, provide sustained energy and are rich in fiber.

Proteins:

Proteins are involved in various bodily functions, including enzyme production, immune system support, and the formation of muscles, skin, and hair. Proteins are essential for the growth, repair, and maintenance of the body tissues. They also contain amino acids, which are the building blocks of proteins. Good sources of protein include meat, poultry, fish, eggs, dairy products, legumes, nuts, and seeds.

Fats:

Fats are an important energy source and help absorb fat-soluble vitamins. Fats are found in foods such as oils, butter, nuts, seeds, avocados, and fatty fish. There are different types of fats, including saturated fats (found in animal products and some plant oils), unsaturated fats (found in plant oils, nuts, and seeds), and trans fats (found in processed and fried foods, and should be limited).

MICRONUTRIENTS

Micronutrients are essential nutrients required by the body in smaller quantities, but they are no less important than macronutrients. They include vitamins and minerals, which play vital roles in various physiological processes and are necessary for overall health and well-being. Micronutrients are crucial for maintaining optimal health, supporting growth and development, and preventing deficiencies or imbalances that can lead to health issues. They work in synergy with macronutrients to ensure the proper functioning of the body's systems. While the body requires them in smaller quantities, their importance should not be underestimated, and a balanced diet that includes a variety of nutrient-rich foods is key to meeting micronutrient needs. In some cases, dietary supplements may be recommended to address specific deficiencies or meet increased requirements.

Micronutrients include vitamins and minerals.

Vitamins:

Vitamins are organic compounds that are crucial for normal growth, development, and metabolism. They support immune function, assist in energy production, and act as antioxidants to protect cells from damage. There are two types of vitamins: water-soluble (B vitamins and vitamin C) and fat-soluble (vitamins A, D, E, and K). Each vitamin plays specific roles in the body and can be obtained from a variety of food sources or supplements.

Minerals:

Minerals are inorganic substances necessary for various bodily functions. They help maintain proper fluid balance, support bone health, assist in nerve function, and contribute to enzyme activity. Examples of minerals include calcium, iron, potassium, magnesium, zinc, and many others. Minerals can be obtained from a diverse range of foods, including fruits, vegetables, dairy products, whole grains, meats, and legumes.

ROLE OF THE FOOD NUTRIENTS IN THE BODY

The foods we eat contain nutrients. Nutrients are substances required by the body to perform its basic functions. Nutrients must be obtained from our diet since the human body can not make them. Nutrients have one or more of three basic functions: they provide energy, contribute to body structure, and/or regulate chemical processes in the body. These basic functions allow us to detect and respond to environmental surroundings, move, excrete wastes, breathe, grow, and reproduce. There are six classes of nutrients required for the body to function and maintain overall health. These are carbohydrates, lipids, proteins, water, vitamins, and minerals. Foods also contain non-nutrient that may be harmful such as natural toxins common in plant foods and additives like some dyes and preservatives or beneficial like antioxidants.

Nutrients plays a crucial roles in the body, supporting various bodily functgions and promoting overall health. Here's a brief explanation of the role of each nutrient and why they are essential:

1.Carbohydrates:

Carbohydrates are the primary source of energy for the body. They are broken down into glucose, which fuels the cells and provides energy for physical activity, brain function, and other metabolic processes. Carbohydrates are also a ready source of energy for the body and provide structural constituents for the formation of cells.

2.Proteins:

Proteins are essential for building and repairing tissues. They are made up of amino acids, which are involved in muscle development, immune system function, enzyme production, and numerous other biological processes. Protein is necessary for tissue formation, cell reparation, and hormone and enzyme production.

3.Fats:

Provides stored energy for the body, it functions as structural components of cells, and signaling molecules for proper cellular communication. It provides insulation to vital organs and works to maintain body temperature. Dietary fats serve as an energy reserve and aid in the absorption of fat-soluble vitamins. They also provide insulation and protection for vital organs. Healthy fats are necessary for cell membrane structure, hormone production, and the absorption of fat-soluble vitamins.

4.Vitamins:

Vitamins are micronutrients that support various bodily functions. They act as coenzymes, assisting enzymes in carrying out chemical reactions. Different vitamins have specific roles, such as vitamin C's involvement in collagen synthesis and vitamin D's role in bone health.

5.Minerals:

Minerals are essential for the body's proper functioning, acting as cofactors for enzymes and participating in various physiological processes. Examples include calcium for bone health, iron for oxygen transport, and potassium for nerve function.

6.Water:

 While not a nutrient, water is vital for survival. It serves as a universal solvent, participates in chemical reactions, regulates body temperature, aids in digestion, transports nutrients and waste, and lubricates joints.

Each nutrient plays a unique role in maintaining good health and ensuring proper bodily functions.

Balanced Meals and Portion Control

Balanced meals and portion control are essential components of maintaining a healthy and well-rounded diet. The concept revolves around ensuring that your meals contain a combination of different food groups in appropriate quantities to meet your nutritional needs while avoiding overeating.

A balanced meal typically consists of three main components: carbohydrates, proteins, and vegetables (or fruits). These components work together to provide a variety of nutrients necessary for optimal functioning of the body. Here's a breakdown of each component:

Carbohydrates: These are the body's primary source of energy. Include whole grains like brown rice, whole wheat bread, or quinoa in your meals. These complex carbohydrates provide fiber, vitamins, and minerals, and help sustain energy levels.

Proteins: Proteins are essential for growth, repair, and maintenance of body tissues. Include lean sources of protein such as poultry, fish, beans, lentils, tofu, or Greek yogurt. These provide important amino acids and help you feel full for longer.

Vegetables (or Fruits): Colorful and nutrient-dense vegetables and fruits should form a significant portion of your meals. They provide essential vitamins, minerals, antioxidants, and fiber. Aim for a variety of colors and types to get a wide range of nutrients.

In addition to balancing the components, portion control is also crucial. It involves consuming appropriate serving sizes to avoid excessive calorie intake. Here are some tips for portion control:

1. Use smaller plates and bowls to create an illusion of a fuller plate, which can help reduce overeating.

2. Listen to your body's hunger and fullness cues. Eat slowly and mindfully, giving your brain enough time to register when you're satisfied.

3. Include appropriate portion sizes of each food group. For example, a palm-sized portion of protein, a fist-sized portion of carbohydrates, and half of your plate filled with vegetables.

4. Be mindful of high-calorie and high-fat foods. Enjoy them in moderation and balance them with healthier choices.

It is important to note that everyone's nutritional needs varies based on factors like age, gender, activity level, and underlying health conditions. It's always beneficial to consult a healthcare professional or a registered dietitian for personalized guidance on balanced meals and portion control that best suit your individual needs.

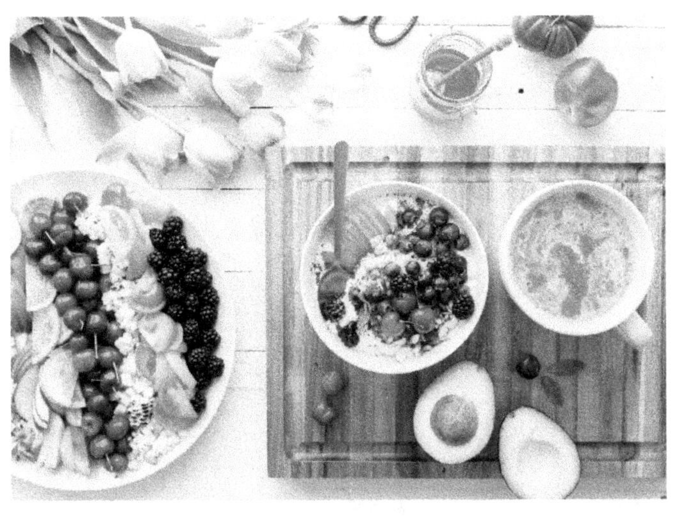

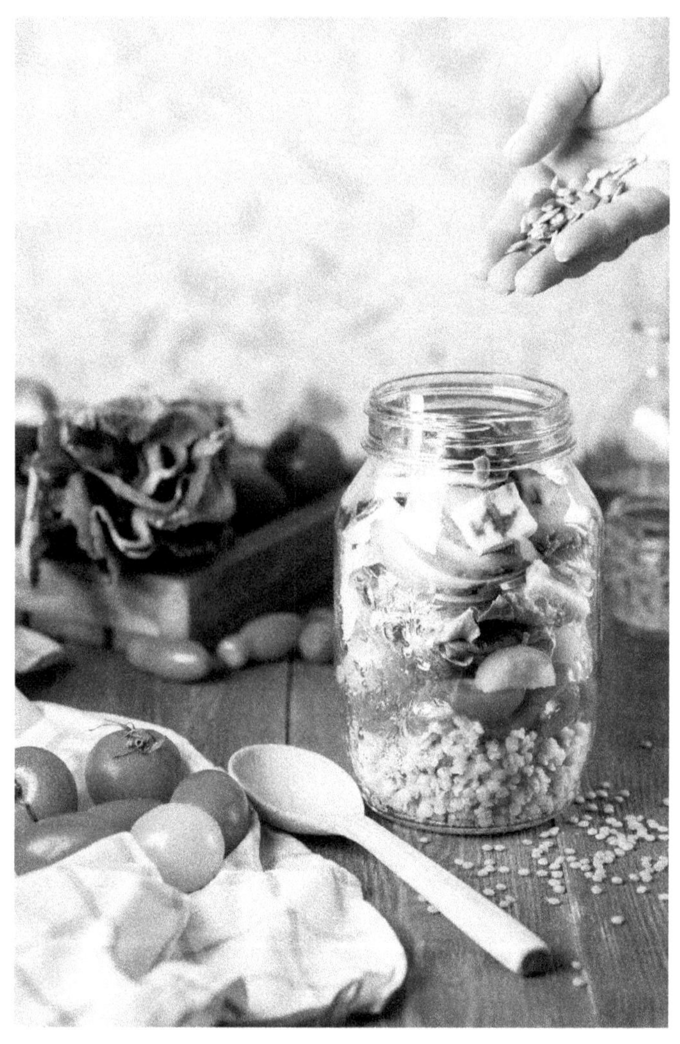

CHAPTER 3:BUILDING HEALTHY PLATE

Building a healthy plate involves selecting a variety of nutritious foods from different food groups to ensure a well-balanced and nutrient-rich meal. Here's a comprehensive guide to creating a healthy plate:

1.Full Half of Your Plate with Vegetables and Fruits:

Aim for a colorful assortment of vegetables and fruits, as they provide essential vitamins, minerals, fiber, and antioxidants.Include a mix of leafy greens, cruciferous vegetables (like broccoli and cauliflower), root vegetables, and a variety of fruits.Opt for fresh, frozen, or canned options without added sugars or excessive sodium.

2.Incorporate Lean Proteins:

Choose lean sources of protein to promote muscle growth and repair, and to keep you feeling full.Options include skinless poultry, fish, beans, lentils, tofu, tempeh, low-fat dairy products, and eggs.Avoid processed meats and opt for grilled, baked, or steamed preparations.

3.Include Whole Grains:

Select whole grains over refined grains to benefit from higher fiber content, vitamins, minerals, and slower digestion.

4.Add Healthy Fats:

Incorporate sources of healthy fats, which are important for brain health and nutrient absorption.Opt for unsaturated fats found in avocados, nuts, seeds, olives, and oils like olive oil or canola oil.Limit saturated and trans fats found in fatty meats, butter, cream, and processed snacks.

5.Moderate Dairy or Dairy Alternatives:

If you consume dairy, choose low-fat or fat-free options like skim milk, yogurt, or cottage cheese.For those avoiding dairy, opt for fortified plant-based milk alternatives like almond milk, soy milk, or oat milk.

6.Stay Hydrated:

Drink water throughout the day to stay hydrated and support bodily functions. Limit sugary beverages like soda and fruit juices, as they often provide empty calories.

7.Minimize Added Sugars and Sodium:

Reduce your consumption of foods high in added sugars and sodium. Check food labels and ingredients lists to identify hidden sources of added sugars and excessive sodium.

This comprehensive guide is a general overview of building a healthy plate. Individual dietary needs may vary, so it's always advisable to consult a registered dietitian or healthcare professional for personalized guidance.

IMPORTANT OF INCORPORATING FRUITS AND VEGETABLES

Incorporating fruits and vegetables into our diet is crucial for maintaining the optimal health and well-being. These nutrient-rich foods offer numerous benefits and should be an essential part of your daily meals. Here's a comprehensive overview of the importance of incorporating fruits and vegetables:

1.Abundance of Essential Nutrients:

Fruits and vegetables provide a wide range of vitamins, including vitamins A, C, E, and K, as well as minerals like potassium and folate. These nutrients support various bodily functions, including immune system function, energy production, cell growth, and maintenance of healthy bones, skin, and eyes.

2.High in Antioxidants:

Fruits and vegetables are rich in antioxidants that help protect the body against free radicals. Free radicals are unstable molecules that can cause cellular damage and contribute to chronic diseases like heart disease, cancer, and neurodegenerative disorders. Antioxidants, such as vitamin C, vitamin E, beta-carotene, and other phytochemicals, neutralize free radicals, reducing the risk of chronic diseases.

3.Fiber for Digestive Health:

Fruits and vegetables are excellent sources of dietary fiber. Fiber promotes healthy digestion by aiding in regular bowel movements, preventing constipation, and maintaining a healthy gut microbiome. It also helps control blood sugar levels, lowers cholesterol levels, and contributes to a feeling of fullness, which can aid in weight management.

4.Disease Prevention:

Consumption of fruits and vegetables helps to reduced the risk of chronic diseases. Research suggests that diets rich in fruits and vegetables may help lower the risk of heart disease, stroke, certain types of cancer (such as colorectal, lung, and stomach cancer), and age-related macular degeneration.

5.Weight Management:

Fruits and vegetables have low calories and are high in fiber, which makes it an excellent choice for weight management. Their high water content and fiber content contribute to a feeling of fullness, reducing the likelihood of overeating. By incorporating fruits and vegetables into your meals, you can increase nutrient density while keeping calorie intake in check.

6.Hydration and Skin Health:

Many fruits and vegetables have high water content, contributing to hydration and overall well-being. Proper hydration is essential for healthy skin, as it helps maintain moisture, elasticity, and a youthful appearance. Certain fruits and vegetables, like berries, citrus fruits, and leafy greens, contain vitamins and antioxidants that promote healthy skin and may help reduce the signs of aging.

7.Versatile and Delicious Options:

Fruits and vegetables offer a wide variety of flavors, textures, and colors, making meals more enjoyable and appealing. You can incorporate them into salads, stir-fries, smoothies, soups, sandwiches, and as snacks. Experimenting with different fruits and vegetables adds variety to your diet, ensuring a wider range of nutrients.

Incorporating a variety of fruits and vegetables into your daily meals is essential for overall health and disease prevention. Strive to consume a rainbow of colors, as different colors indicate different nutrient profiles. Remember to choose fresh, seasonal produce whenever possible and aim for a balance between raw and cooked options to maximize nutrient intake.

CHOOSING WHOLE GRAINS OVER REFINED GRAINS

Choosing whole grains over refined grains is a wise and health-conscious decision that can have significant benefits for your overall well-being. Whole grains are less processed and retain their nutrient-rich components, making them a superior choice compared to refined grains. Here's a comprehensive overview of why you should opt for whole grains:

1.Higher Nutritional Value:

Whole grains contain all parts of the grain kernel—the bran, germ, and endosperm—retaining essential nutrients. They are rich in dietary fiber, B vitamins (such as thiamin, riboflavin, niacin, and folate), minerals (such as magnesium, selenium, and zinc), and phytochemicals. These nutrients contribute to various bodily functions, including energy production, digestion, heart health, and immune function.

2.Dietary Fiber Content:

Whole grains are an excellent source of dietary fiber, which plays a vital role in maintaining a healthy digestive system. Fiber helps prevent constipation, promotes regular bowel movements, and supports the growth of beneficial gut bacteria. Adequate fiber intake has been associated with a reduced risk of heart disease, type 2 diabetes, and certain types of cancer.

3.Slower Digestion and Sustained Energy:

Whole grains have a lower glycemic index compared to refined grains, meaning they are digested and absorbed more slowly. This slower digestion results in a gradual release of glucose into the bloodstream, providing sustained energy and preventing blood sugar spikes and crashes. Choosing whole grains can help regulate blood sugar levels and may reduce the risk of developing type 2 diabetes.

4.Heart Health Benefits:

Whole grains have been linked to a lower risk of heart disease and improved cardiovascular health. The fiber, antioxidants, and phytochemicals found in whole grains work together to reduce inflammation, lower LDL (bad) cholesterol levels, and maintain healthy blood pressure. Consuming whole grains as part of a heart-healthy diet may help protect against heart disease and stroke.

5.Weight Management and Satiety:

Whole grains are more filling and can contribute to a sense of fullness, which aids in weight management. The combination of fiber, protein, and complex carbohydrates in whole grains helps you feel satisfied for longer, reducing the likelihood of overeating. Choosing whole grains over refined grains can support healthy weight maintenance and help prevent excessive calorie consumption.

6.Versatility in Cooking:

Whole grains offer a wide range of options to incorporate into your meals. Examples of whole grains include whole wheat, oats, brown rice, quinoa, barley, buckwheat, and millet. You can use them as the base for pilafs, salads, soups, stir-fries, and side dishes, or incorporate them into baked goods and breakfast cereals.

When selecting whole grains, be mindful of food labels and ingredient lists. Look for products that explicitly state "100% whole grain" or have whole grains listed as the first ingredient. Be cautious of terms like "multigrain" or "wheat" since they may still contain refined grains. By choosing whole grains as the foundation of your diet, you can enjoy their nutritional benefits and contribute to your long-term health and well-being.

IMPORTANT OF INCLUDING LEAN PROTEINS AND PLANT-BASED PROTEIN SOURCE

Incorporating lean proteins and plant-based protein sources into your diet provides a balanced intake of essential amino acids and vital nutrients. Whether you choose lean animal proteins or opt for plant-based options, diversifying your protein sources promotes a well-rounded and sustainable approach to nutrition. Including lean proteins and plant-based protein sources in your diet is essential for overall health and well-being. Proteins plays an important role in building and repairing body tissues, supporting immune function, and providing energy. Here's a comprehensive overview of why you should incorporate lean proteins and plant-based protein sources into your meals:

Lean Proteins

1.Muscle Growth and Repair:

Lean protein sources, such as skinless poultry, fish, lean cuts of beef, and low-fat dairy products, provide essential amino acids necessary for muscle growth and repair. They contain high-quality protein with a balanced amino acid profile, which supports the maintenance and development of lean muscle mass.

2.Satiety and Weight Management:

Protein is known for its ability to promote feelings of fullness and satiety. Including lean protein in your meals helps control hunger, reduce cravings, and prevent overeating, which can aid in weight management and weight loss efforts.

3.Nutrient Density:

Lean protein sources often come with additional nutrients, such as vitamins, minerals, and healthy fats. For example, fish is a rich source of omega-3 fatty acids, while lean cuts of beef and poultry provide iron, zinc, and B vitamins. Choosing lean protein options allows you to obtain these beneficial nutrients while keeping saturated fat intake in check.

4.Heart Health:

Lean proteins are generally lower in saturated fat compared to fatty cuts of meat or processed meats. A diet rich in lean proteins has been associated with a reduced risk of heart disease, as it helps maintain healthy cholesterol levels and blood pressure.

Plant-Based Protein Sources:

1.Nutrient-Rich Options:

Plant-based protein sources, such as legumes (beans, lentils, and chickpeas), tofu, tempeh, seitan, quinoa, nuts, and seeds, offer a wide array of essential nutrients. These sources provide protein, fiber, healthy fats, vitamins, minerals, and antioxidants that are beneficial for overall health.

2.Heart-Healthy Profile:

Plant-based protein sources are typically low in saturated fat and cholesterol, making them heart-healthy choices. They also often contain unsaturated fats, including omega-3 fatty acids, which support cardiovascular health.

3.Fiber Content:

Many plant-based protein sources are rich in dietary fiber, which promotes healthy digestion, helps regulate blood sugar levels, and contributes to a feeling of fullness.

Legumes, in particular, are excellent sources of both protein and fiber, making them a valuable addition to a plant-based diet.

4.Reduced Environmental Impact:

Choosing plant-based protein sources can have a positive impact on the environment.

Plant-based proteins require fewer resources, such as land, water, and energy, compared to animal-based proteins, leading to lower greenhouse gas emissions and reduced strain on natural resources.

5.Variety and Culinary Flexibility:

Plant-based protein sources offer versatility in cooking, allowing for a wide range of delicious and creative dishes. You can experiment with plant-based proteins in stir-fries, salads, soups, curries, grain bowls, and plant-based meat alternatives.

INCORPORATING HEALTHY FATS

It's important to note that while healthy fats are beneficial, moderation is key. They are calorie-dense, so portion control is necessary to maintain a balanced diet. Incorporate sources of healthy fats into your meals, such as avocados, nuts, seeds, fatty fish, olive oil, and coconut oil, while being mindful of overall calorie intake and individual dietary needs. Consulting with a healthcare professional or registered dietitian can provide personalized guidance on incorporating healthy fats into your specific diet plan.

TIPS FOR REDUCING ADDED SUGARS AND SODIUM INTAKE

Reducing added sugars and sodium intake is a wise choice for promoting overall health and well-being. Here are some tips to help you accomplish this:

Read food labels:

Start by checking the nutrition labels on packaged foods. Look for the amounts of added sugars and sodium per serving. Ingredients are listed in descending order, so if sugar or sodium appears near the top, it indicates a higher content.

Choose whole unprocessed foods:

Opt for whole foods like fresh fruits, vegetables, lean meats, fish, whole grains, and legumes. These foods are naturally low in added sugars and sodium. By cooking meals from scratch, you have better control over the ingredients and can minimize added sugars and sodium.

Limit sugary beverages:

Sugary drinks like soda, sweetened juices, and energy drinks are significant sources of added sugars. Choose water, unsweetened tea, or naturally flavored water instead. If you crave sweetness, try infusing water with fruits or adding a splash of citrus juice.

Be mindful of condiments and sauces:

Many condiments and sauces, such as ketchup, barbecue sauce, salad dressings, and soy sauce, can be high in added sugars and sodium. Check the labels for lower-sugar and lower-sodium alternatives, or consider making your own healthier versions at home.

Reduce processed and packaged snacks:

Processed and packaged snacks like cookies, cakes, chips, and pretzels often contain high amounts of added sugars and sodium. Look for healthier snack options like fresh fruits, raw nuts, seeds, or homemade snacks with natural ingredients.

Cook at home:

Preparing meals at home gives you better control over the ingredients you use. Use herbs, spices, and other flavorings to enhance the taste of your meals without relying on excessive sodium. Experiment with different cooking techniques to bring out the natural flavors of ingredients.

Be cautious of hidden sugars and sodium:

Added sugars and sodium can hide in surprising places like canned soups, salad dressings, cereals, and even seemingly healthy foods like yogurt and granola bars. Always check the labels and choose options with lower amounts of added sugars and sodium.

Gradually reduce intake:

Making drastic changes to your diet can be challenging. Start by gradually reducing your intake of added sugars and sodium. Small, sustainable changes over time can make a big difference in the long run.

Remember that it's important to listen to your body and find the approach that works best for you. If you have any specific health concerns or dietary restrictions, it's always a good idea to consult with a healthcare professional or registered dietitian for personalized advice and guidance.

CHAPTER 4: MEAL PLANNING AND PREPARATION

Meal planning is the process of organizing and preparing meals in advance. It involves deciding what to eat, creating a menu, and outlining a grocery list to ensure you have the necessary ingredients on hand. Meal planning can be done on a weekly, bi-weekly, or monthly basis, depending on individual preferences and needs.Meal planning can be as simple or as detailed as you prefer. It can involve designing a full week of meals, including breakfast, lunch, dinner, and snacks, or focusing on specific meals that pose challenges. The key is to find a system that works for you and helps you achieve your goals while maintaining flexibility and enjoyment in your meals.

Meal planning plays a crucial role in maintaining a healthy diet with the following reasons:

1.Nutritional balance:

Meal planning allows you to ensure that your meals are well-balanced and provide a variety of nutrients. By intentionally including fruits, vegetables, whole grains, lean proteins, and healthy fats in your meal plans, you can meet your body's nutritional needs and support overall health.

2.Portion control:

Planning your meals in advance helps with portion control, preventing overeating and promoting healthy portion sizes. When you have pre-determined meals and servings, you're less likely to indulge in oversized portions or reach for unhealthy snacks.

3.Healthy ingredient choices:

When you plan your meals, you have the opportunity to select fresh, whole ingredients and avoid processed foods that are often high in unhealthy additives, preservatives, sugars, and unhealthy fats. This allows you to prioritize nutrient-dense foods that nourish your body.

4.Weight management:

Meal planning can be an effective tool for weight management. By carefully considering the calorie content of your meals and controlling portion sizes, you can create a calorie deficit for weight loss or maintain a healthy weight. Additionally, having a clear meal plan reduces impulsive food choices that may hinder your weight management goals.

5.Time and convenience:

Meal planning can save you time and make healthy eating more convenient. By prepping ingredients in advance, you can streamline cooking and reduce the time spent on meal preparation during busy weekdays. This can help you avoid resorting to unhealthy fast food or takeout options when you're short on time or energy.

6.Financial savings:

Planning your meals in advance allows you to create a shopping list based on your planned recipes, which helps you avoid impulse purchases and food waste. By making a list and sticking to it, you can optimize your grocery shopping and reduce unnecessary spending. Moreover, preparing meals at home is generally more cost-effective than dining out.

7.Reduce decision fatigue:

Meal planning eliminates the daily stress of deciding what to eat, especially when hunger strikes or time is limited. Having a set plan reduces decision fatigue and helps you make healthier choices without succumbing to less nutritious options.

8.Dietary adherence:

If you have specific dietary goals or restrictions, such as following a specific diet plan (e.g., Mediterranean, vegetarian, or ketogenic), managing a health condition, or addressing food allergies or intolerances, meal planning can provide structure and support to help you adhere to your dietary requirements.

By incorporating meal planning into your daily routine, you can establish healthier eating habits, optimize your nutrient intake, save time and money, and support your overall well-being. Remember to personalize your meal plans to meet your specific needs and consult with a healthcare professional or registered dietitian for personalized advice and guidance.

TIPS FOR A WELL-BALANCED MEAL PLAN

Creating a well-balanced meal plan involves considering various aspects of nutrition and ensuring that your meals provide a good balance of essential nutrients. Here are 10 tips to help you create a well-balanced meal plan:

1.Include a variety of food groups:

Always aim to include foods from all major food groups in your meal plan, including fruits, vegetables, whole grains, lean proteins, and healthy fats. Each food group provides unique nutrients, so incorporating a variety of foods helps ensure a diverse nutrient intake.

2.Prioritize fruits and vegetables:

Always include a generous portion of fruits and vegetables in your meal plan. They are rich in vitamins, minerals, antioxidants, and fiber. Try to incorporate a variety of colorful options to maximize nutrient diversity.

3.Opt for whole grains:

Choose whole grains over refined grains whenever possible. Whole grains such as brown rice, quinoa, whole wheat bread, and oats provide more fiber, vitamins, and minerals than their refined counterparts.

4.Include lean proteins:

Incorporate lean protein sources into your meals, such as skinless poultry, fish, legumes, tofu, and low-fat dairy products. Proteins are essential for muscle repair, satiety, and overall health.

5.Incorporate healthy fats:

Always add some sources of healthy fats like avocados, nuts, seeds, olive oil, and fatty fish (e.g., salmon, mackerel) in your meal plan. Healthy fats provide essential fatty acids and help with nutrient absorption.

6.Monitor portion sizes:

Try placing attention to portion sizes to avoid overeating. Use visual cues, measuring tools, or portion control containers to help you estimate appropriate serving sizes.

7.Control added sugars and sodium:

Limit the intake of foods and beverages high in added sugars and sodium. Choose minimally processed options and read food labels to make informed choices. Opt for natural sources of sweetness, such as fresh fruits, instead of sugary snacks or desserts.

8.Plan for snacks:

Don't forget to include healthy snacks in your meal plan. Opt for options like raw nuts, fresh fruit, yogurt, vegetable sticks with hummus, or homemade energy bars to keep you satisfied between meals.

9.Drink plenty of water:

Hydration is essential for overall health. Always include water as your primary beverage throughout the day and limit sugary drinks and excessive caffeine intake.

10.Consider individual needs and preferences:

Customize your meal plan based on your individual needs, preferences, and any dietary restrictions or allergies you may have. Seek guidance from a healthcare professional or registered dietitian for personalized advice.

Remember that meal planning should be flexible and adaptable to your lifestyle. Experiment with different recipes, flavors, and cooking methods to keep your meals interesting and enjoyable. Regularly review and adjust your meal plan to accommodate changes in your routine, seasonal produce, and personal goals.

MEAL PREPPING AND BATCH COOKING

Meal prepping refers to the practice of planning, preparing, and packaging meals in advance, typically for a specific period, such as a week. It involves cooking and assembling portions of meals ahead of time, which can then be conveniently stored and reheated when needed. The purpose of meal prepping is to save time and effort during busy weekdays, ensure healthier eating habits, and have more control over the nutritional content and portion sizes of meals. It allows individuals to make deliberate food choices, reduce reliance on takeout or processed foods, and promotes consistency in maintaining a well-balanced diet.

Meal prepping and batch cooking can be great for convenience and saving time in the kitchen. Meal prepping and batch cooking are flexible, and you can adjust the process to suit your needs. It's a great way to save time, reduce stress, and ensure you have nutritious meals ready to go throughout the week.

Here's a simple guide to help you get started:

Plan your meals:

Decide which meals you want to prep for the week. Consider breakfast, lunch, dinner, and snacks. Make a list of the recipes and ingredients you'll need.

Grocery shopping:

Go shopping with your list to ensure you have all the necessary ingredients. Buying in bulk can be cost-effective for batch cooking.

Prep ingredients:

Once you're back home, wash, chop, and prepare your ingredients. This can include cutting vegetables, marinating meats, or cooking grains. Having ingredients prepped in advance saves time during the week.

Cook in batches:

Choose a day or two when you have some free time and cook large quantities of certain dishes. For example, you could make a big pot of chili, a tray of roasted vegetables, or a batch of grilled chicken breasts. Divide these cooked items into individual portions or family-sized portions.

Storage:

Use airtight containers or meal prep containers to store your prepared meals. Label them with the contents and date to keep track of freshness. Stack them in the fridge or freezer, depending on when you plan to consume them.

Portion control:

If you're aiming for specific portion sizes, use a food scale or measuring cups to divide the meals evenly. This helps maintain a balanced diet and saves time when grabbing a meal on busy days.

Variety and customization:

Consider making a variety of dishes, so you don't get bored. Prepare different proteins, vegetables, grains, and sauces, allowing you to mix and match throughout the week. Customize the flavors and seasonings according to your preferences.

Reheating:

When it's time to eat, simply reheat your prepped meals. Microwave or oven methods work well, depending on the dish. Add fresh toppings or sauces to enhance the flavors.

GROCERY SHOPPING FOR HEALTHY FOODS INGREDIENTS

Grocery shopping is the act of purchasing food, beverages, household supplies, and other items from a grocery store or supermarket. It involves making a list of needed items, visiting the store, selecting products from the shelves or refrigerated sections, and proceeding to the checkout to pay for the items. Grocery shopping is an essential task for stocking up on groceries and household necessities, ensuring that you have the ingredients and supplies you need for cooking, eating, and maintaining your home. It can be done in physical stores or, in some cases, online through e-commerce platforms that offer grocery delivery or pickup services.

Establishing a habit of mindful grocery shopping and consistently selecting nutritious ingredients can contribute to a healthier diet and overall well-being. Here are some strategies for grocery shopping to help you choose healthy ingredients:

1.Make a list: Plan your meals in advance and create a shopping list based on those recipes. This helps you stay focused and avoid impulse purchases of unhealthy items.

2. Shop the perimeter: The outer aisles of the grocery store often contain fresh produce, lean proteins, dairy, and whole grains. Spend more time in these areas to fill your cart with nutritious options.

3. Choose fresh produce: Opt for a variety of colorful fruits and vegetables. Look for items that are in season for the best flavor and nutritional value.

4. Read labels: When buying packaged foods, read the nutrition labels carefully. Look for products with minimal additives, lower sodium content, and limited added sugars. Pay attention to serving sizes to understand the true nutritional values.

5. Go for whole grains: Select whole grain options like whole wheat bread, brown rice, and whole grain cereals. These contain more fiber and nutrients compared to refined grains.

6. Select lean proteins: Choose lean cuts of meat, such as skinless poultry, fish, or lean beef. Incorporate plant-based proteins like legumes, tofu, or tempeh into your shopping as well.

7. Limit processed foods: Minimize your intake of highly processed foods, including snacks, sugary drinks, and pre-packaged meals.

These tend to be higher in unhealthy fats, added sugars, and sodium.

8. Check for sales and discounts:

Keep an eye out for sales and discounts on healthy items. This can help you save money while still purchasing nutritious ingredients.

9. Don't shop on an empty stomach: Eat a balanced meal or snack before going grocery shopping. Shopping when hungry can lead to impulsive choices and the temptation to buy less healthy options.

10. Stick to your list: Stay disciplined and avoid deviating from your shopping list. This helps you avoid buying unnecessary items and keeps your focus on healthier choices.

CHAPTER 5: HEALTHY COOKING TECHNIQUES

Healthier cooking methods refer to techniques and practices that retain the nutritional value of food while minimizing the use of unhealthy ingredients or cooking techniques. These methods prioritize the preservation of vitamins, minerals, and other beneficial components of ingredients, while reducing the intake of excessive fats, salt, and added sugars. Some examples of healthier cooking methods include steaming, boiling, grilling, roasting, baking, and sautéing with minimal oil. These methods help to maintain the natural flavors and textures of the food, making it both nutritious and delicious.

Cooking is not only about creating delicious meals; it also plays a crucial role in maintaining our health and well-being. When it comes to preparing meals, choosing healthier cooking methods can significantly impact the nutritional value of the food we consume. In this introduction, we will explore some popular healthier cooking methods, namely grilling, baking, steaming, and sautéing, and how they contribute to a healthier lifestyle.

Grilling:

Grilling is a cooking method that involves the application of dry heat directly to the food. It is often associated with outdoor barbecues and imparts a unique smoky flavor to various ingredients. Grilling is an excellent choice for reducing the amount of added fats, as it allows excess fats to drip away from the food. It also helps retain the natural flavors and nutrients present in the ingredients.

Baking:

Baking is a method that utilizes dry heat in an enclosed space, such as an oven, to cook food. It is widely used for preparing bread, pastries, and a variety of dishes. Baking generally requires less oil or fat compared to frying or sautéing, making it a healthier option. It helps to preserve the nutrients and flavors of ingredients while creating appealing textures through gentle and controlled heat.

Steaming:

Steaming is a cooking technique that involves cooking food by exposing it to steam, either in a steamer or by using other equipment like a microwave or stovetop. Steaming is a gentle and moisture-rich method that retains the natural colors, textures, and nutrients of the food. It requires minimal or no added fats, making it an ideal choice for those aiming to reduce calorie intake.

Sautéing:

Sautéing is a quick cooking method that involves frying ingredients in a small amount of oil or fat over high heat. While it may not be as low in fat as steaming or baking, sautéing allows for precise control over the amount of oil used. By using heart-healthy oils and incorporating a variety of vegetables, lean proteins, and whole grains, sautéing can be a nutritious cooking method that adds vibrant flavors to your dishes.

By incorporating these healthier cooking methods into your culinary repertoire, you can enhance the nutritional profile of your meals while still enjoying delicious flavors. Always try to prioritize fresh and wholesome ingredients, use minimal unhealthy fats, and be mindful of portion sizes to promote a balanced and healthy lifestyle.

EFFECT OF UNHEALTHY COOKING OS AND EXCESSIVE FRAYING

It's important to note that occasional consumption of fried foods is unlikely to cause severe health issues. However, to promote better health, it's recommended to limit the use of unhealthy cooking oils and reduce excessive frying. By choosing healthier cooking methods and using oils with better nutritional profiles, you can minimize the potential negative effects on your health. Using unhealthy cooking oils and excessive frying can have various negative effects on your health.

Reducing the use of unhealthy cooking oils and excessive frying can greatly contribute to a healthier diet. While it's important to reduce the use of unhealthy cooking oils and excessive frying, it's also okay to enjoy your favorite indulgent foods occasionally. By incorporating these tips into your cooking routine, you can make gradual and sustainable changes towards a healthier approach in the kitchen. Here are some tips to help you achieve that:

1.Choose healthier cooking oils:

Opt for oils that are high in unsaturated fats, such as olive oil, avocado oil, or canola oil. These oils contain healthier fats compared to saturated or trans fats, which are typically found in butter or solid fats like shortening.

2.Use oil sparingly:

Instead of pouring oil directly into the pan, try using cooking spray or a brush to lightly coat the surface. This helps reduce the amount of oil used while still providing enough lubrication to prevent sticking.

3.Experiment with alternative cooking methods:

Explore cooking methods that require less or no oil at all. Steaming, grilling, baking, or broiling are great alternatives that can preserve the flavors and nutrients of your food without the need for excessive frying.

4.Bake or roast instead of frying:

When preparing dishes like chicken or fish, consider baking or roasting them in the oven instead of deep-frying. This method can achieve a crispy texture without the added oil.

5.Use non-stick cookware: Non-stick pans and pots require less oil or fat to prevent sticking. This allows you to sauté or cook with minimal oil while still achieving desirable results.

6.Opt for healthier cooking techniques: Explore methods like stir-frying, steaming, poaching, or boiling, which require minimal oil. These techniques can help you achieve flavorful and nutritious meals with reduced reliance on unhealthy fats.

7.Drain excess oil: After cooking, use paper towels or a slotted spoon to remove any excess oil from fried foods. This can help reduce the overall fat content of the dish.

8.Enhance flavors with herbs and spices: Instead of relying solely on oil for flavor, experiment with herbs, spices, and seasonings to add taste to your dishes. This allows you to reduce the amount of oil used without compromising on flavor.

HEALTHY INGREDIENTS SUBSTITUTES FOR TRADITIONAL RECIPES

To adjust quantities and cooking times as needed when making substitutions for some recipes, as they can sometimes alter the texture and taste of the final dish. Here are some healthy ingredient substitutions you can consider for traditional recipes:

1.Replace butter or margarine with mashed avocado, unsweetened applesauce, or Greek yogurt to reduce saturated fat.

2.Substitute refined white flour with whole wheat flour, almond flour, or oat flour for added fiber and nutrients.

3.Use natural sweeteners like honey, maple syrup, or mashed bananas instead of refined sugar in baked goods.

4.Swap full-fat dairy products with low-fat or skim versions, such as using skim milk instead of whole milk.

5.Opt for lean proteins like skinless chicken breast, turkey, or tofu instead of fatty cuts of meat.

6.Replace regular pasta with whole wheat pasta, brown rice, or zucchini noodles (zoodles) for a healthier alternative.

7.Use herbs and spices instead of excessive salt to enhance the flavor of your dishes and reduce sodium intake.

8.Incorporate a variety of vegetables into your recipes, such as spinach, kale, or zucchini, to boost nutritional value.

9.Choose healthier cooking methods like baking, grilling, or steaming instead of frying to reduce added fats.

10.Use unsweetened almond milk or coconut milk as a dairy-free alternative in recipes that call for regular milk.

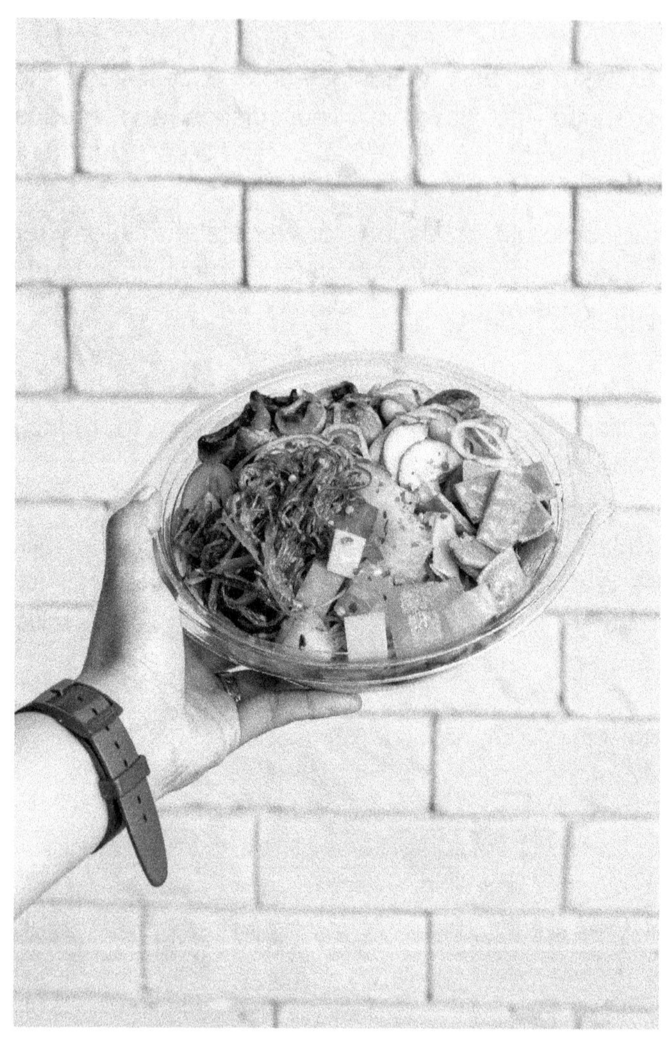

CHAPTER 6: SMART SNACKING AND HYDRATION

Smart snacking refers to the practice of making healthy and mindful choices when it comes to snacks. It involves selecting nutritious options that provide energy and essential nutrients while avoiding excessive calories, added sugars, and unhealthy fats. Examples of smart snacks include fruits, vegetables, nuts, yogurt, and whole-grain crackers.

Hydration, on the other hand, refers to maintaining adequate fluid levels in the body. Staying properly hydrated is essential for overall health and well-being. It helps regulate body temperature, supports digestion, lubricates joints, and enables various bodily functions. Drinking water is the most common way to hydrate, but other beverages like herbal tea, unsweetened fruit juices, and low-fat milk can also contribute to hydration.

Snacking has become an integral part of our modern lifestyle, but not all snacks are created equal. The choices we make when selecting our snacks can have a significant impact on our health and well-being. Opting for nutrient-dense snacks over processed snacks is a smart choice that can transform your snacking habits and support a healthier diet. Here's why and how you should choose nutrient-dense snacks:

What are Nutrient-Dense Snacks?

Nutrient-dense snacks are foods that provide a high concentration of essential nutrients, such as vitamins, minerals, fiber, and antioxidants, relative to their caloric content. These snacks offer a plethora of health benefits while being lower in added sugars, unhealthy fats, and artificial additives compared to processed snacks.

The Benefits of Nutrient-Dense Snacks:

a. Sustained Energy: Nutrient-dense snacks contain complex carbohydrates, healthy fats, and protein, which provide sustained energy levels, keeping you feeling full and satisfied for longer periods. This can help prevent energy crashes and the subsequent cravings for unhealthy foods.

b. Essential Nutrients: Nutrient-dense snacks offer a wide range of essential vitamins, minerals, and antioxidants that support overall health and well-being. They contribute to a stronger immune system, improved digestion, enhanced brain function, and better overall nutrition.

c. Weight Management: Nutrient-dense snacks can aid in weight management. Their high fiber content promotes feelings of fullness and helps control appetite, reducing the likelihood of overeating. Additionally, these snacks tend to be lower in calories while providing greater satiety, making them an effective tool for weight control.

d. Disease Prevention: Regularly consuming nutrient-dense snacks can help reduce the risk of chronic diseases, including heart disease, type 2 diabetes, and certain types of cancer. The abundance of vitamins, minerals, and antioxidants in these snacks supports a healthy immune system and helps protect against oxidative stress and inflammation.

Tips for Choosing Nutrient-Dense Snacks:

a. Whole Foods: Opt for snacks that are made from whole, unprocessed ingredients. Fresh fruits and vegetables, raw or roasted nuts and seeds, whole grains, and legumes are excellent choices. These foods are naturally nutrient-dense and provide a range of health benefits.

b. Minimize Processed Snacks: Limit your intake of processed snacks such as chips, cookies, and candy, as they are often high in added sugars, unhealthy fats, and empty calories. These snacks provide little nutritional value and can contribute to weight gain and health problems.

c. Snack Preparation: Prepare your own nutrient-dense snacks at home to have healthier options readily available. Cut up fruits and vegetables, portion out trail mixes or homemade granola, or make your own energy balls using nutritious ingredients. This way, you have control over the quality of ingredients and can tailor your snacks to your preferences.

d. Portion Control: While nutrient-dense snacks are healthier choices, portion control is still important. Even healthy snacks can contribute to weight gain if consumed excessively. Pay attention to serving sizes and aim for a balanced intake.

By choosing nutrient-dense snacks over processed options, you can transform your snacking habits into a powerful tool for better health. These snacks provide essential nutrients, sustained energy, weight management support, and disease prevention benefits. Embrace nutrient-dense snacking as a key component of your overall healthy eating plan and enjoy the positive impact it can have on your well-being.

HEALTHY AND SATISFYING SNACK OPTIONS IDEAS

Snacking can be a great way to keep your energy levels up and satisfy hunger between meals. However, it's important to choose snacks that are both healthy and satisfying. Here are some ideas for nutritious and delicious snack options that will leave you feeling nourished and satisfied:

1.Fresh Fruit: Enjoy a variety of fresh fruits like apples, bananas, oranges, berries, or grapes. They are packed with vitamins, minerals, and fiber, and provide a refreshing and naturally sweet snack.

2.Veggie Sticks with Hummus: Slice up crunchy vegetables such as carrots, celery, bell peppers, and cucumbers. Pair them with a serving of hummus for a satisfying combination of fiber, vitamins, and plant-based protein.

3.Greek Yogurt with Berries: Choose a plain Greek yogurt and top it with fresh berries like strawberries, blueberries, or raspberries. Greek yogurt is high in protein, while the berries add a burst of antioxidants and natural sweetness.

4.Nuts and Seeds: Opt for a handful of unsalted nuts and seeds, such as almonds, walnuts, pumpkin seeds, or sunflower seeds. They provide healthy fats, protein, and essential minerals.

5.Whole Grain Crackers with Nut Butter: Choose whole grain crackers or rice cakes and spread them with a natural nut butter like almond or peanut butter. This combination offers a balance of carbohydrates, protein, and healthy fats.

6.Hard-Boiled Eggs: Hard-boiled eggs are a convenient and protein-rich snack. They are packed with essential amino acids and can help keep you feeling full and satisfied.

7.Avocado Toast: Top a slice of whole grain bread with mashed avocado. Sprinkle some sea salt, black pepper, and a squeeze of lemon juice for a delicious and nutritious snack.

8.Homemade Trail Mix: Create your own trail mix by combining a variety of nuts, seeds, and dried fruits. Customize it to your liking with options like almonds, cashews, pumpkin seeds, dried cranberries, or unsweetened coconut flakes.

9.Smoothie: Blend together a combination of fruits, vegetables, and a liquid base like almond milk or coconut water to create a refreshing and nutritious smoothie. You can also add protein powder or Greek yogurt for an extra protein boost.

10.Roasted Chickpeas: Drain and rinse a can of chickpeas, then toss them in olive oil, salt, and spices of your choice. Roast them in the oven until crispy for a fiber-rich and flavorful snack.

It is important to listen to your body's hunger and fullness cues, and choose snacks that align with your dietary preferences and nutritional needs. These ideas can serve as a starting point for healthy and satisfying snack options, allowing you to enjoy delicious flavors while nourishing your body.

IMPORTANT OF STAYING HYDRATED

Staying properly hydrated is essential for maintaining overall health and well-being. Water plays a crucial role in numerous bodily functions and provides a range of benefits. Here's why hydration is important and some practical tips to help you drink more water:

1. Importance of Hydration:

Regulates Body Temperature: Water helps regulate body temperature by releasing heat through sweat. It prevents overheating during physical activity or in hot environments.

Supports Digestion: Sufficient hydration aids in digestion, as water helps break down food and supports the absorption of nutrients. It also helps prevent constipation by promoting regular bowel movements.

Lubricates Joints: Adequate hydration helps lubricate joints and cushions tissues, promoting smooth movement and reducing the risk of joint pain or discomfort.

Enhances Cognitive Function: The brain relies on proper hydration to function optimally. Staying hydrated can improve concentration, focus, and mental clarity.

Supports Kidney Function: Water is crucial for kidney function, as it helps flush out waste products and toxins from the body. It plays a vital role in maintaining optimal kidney health.

2. Tips for Drinking More Water:

Carry a Water Bottle: Keep a reusable water bottle with you throughout the day. This serves as a reminder to drink water regularly and makes it easily accessible.

Set Reminders: Use phone alarms or reminders to prompt yourself to drink water at regular intervals. This can help establish a hydration routine.

Infuse with Flavor: If plain water is unappealing, infuse it with natural flavors. Add slices of lemon, cucumber, mint leaves, or berries to your water for a refreshing taste.

Make it Accessible: Place water in visible and convenient locations, such as your desk, kitchen counter, or car cup holder. Having water within reach makes it more likely that you'll drink it.

Create Goals: Set daily water intake goals. Aim to drink a certain number of cups or ounces throughout the day and track your progress. This can provide motivation and help you stay on track.

Use Apps or Trackers: Use smartphone apps or wearable devices that track your water intake. These tools can provide reminders, monitor your hydration, and help you stay accountable.
G. Drink Before Meals: Make it a habit to drink a glass of water before each meal. Not only does this

contribute to your daily water intake, but it can also help with portion control and digestion.

Herbal Teas and Infusions: Enjoy herbal teas or infusions as a way to increase your fluid intake. These beverages are hydrating and offer a variety of flavors and health benefits.

Eat Hydrating Foods: Incorporate foods with high water content into your diet. Cucumbers, watermelon, oranges, and celery are examples of hydrating foods that can contribute to your overall hydration.

It is important to note that needs for water by individuals varies depending on factors such as activity level, climate, and overall health. Pay attention to your body's thirst cues and aim to drink water consistently throughout the day. By following these tips, you can develop healthy hydration habits and ensure you're staying adequately hydrated for optimal health.

CHAPTER 7: MINDFUL EATING

Mindful eating is a practice that involves bringing awareness and attention to the entire eating experience, from food selection to consumption. It focuses on cultivating a non-judgmental and present-moment awareness of one's thoughts, feelings, and sensations related to eating. By engaging in mindful eating, individuals can develop a healthier relationship with food and experience a range of benefits. By practicing mindful eating, individuals can cultivate a more balanced and harmonious relationship with food. The benefits extend beyond nutrition, encompassing psychological, emotional, and physical aspects of well-being. Mindful eating can contribute to a healthier lifestyle, improved digestion, weight management, and a positive mindset towards food and eating. Here's a well-explained overview of the concept of mindful eating and its advantages:

1. Bringing Awareness: Mindful eating encourages individuals to become more aware of their eating habits, including the reasons for eating, hunger and fullness cues, and the sensations and flavors of food. It brings attention to the present moment, fostering a deeper connection with the act of eating.

2. Embracing Non-judgment: Mindful eating emphasizes a non-judgmental attitude towards food choices and eating behaviors. It helps individuals let go of self-criticism and guilt, allowing for a more positive and compassionate approach to nourishing the body.

3. Slowing Down and Enjoying Food: Mindful eating promotes a slower pace of eating, allowing individuals to savor each bite and fully experience the taste, texture, and aroma of food. By slowing down, people can better recognize their satiety and avoid overeating.

4. Recognizing Hunger and Fullness: Mindful eating encourages individuals to tune in to their body's hunger and fullness cues. This awareness helps prevent both undereating and overeating, as individuals learn to eat in response to physiological hunger and stop when they feel comfortably satisfied.

5. Enhanced Digestion: By eating mindfully and chewing food thoroughly, the digestive process is optimized. Chewing food well helps break it down into smaller particles, aiding digestion and nutrient absorption. It can also reduce digestive discomfort, such as bloating or indigestion.

6. Emotional Regulation: Mindful eating provides an opportunity to explore the emotional and psychological aspects of eating. It encourages individuals to recognize and understand emotional triggers for eating, helping them differentiate between physical and emotional hunger. This awareness supports healthier coping mechanisms for managing emotions.

7. Weight Management: Mindful eating can be a valuable tool for weight management. By paying attention to hunger and fullness cues, individuals are more likely to eat in response to true physiological hunger rather than emotional or environmental triggers. This can lead to improved portion control and a better balance between energy intake and expenditure.

8. Improved Food Choices: Mindful eating promotes a greater connection with the body's needs, leading to more conscious and intentional food choices. Individuals are more likely to select nourishing foods that support their well-being rather than relying on impulsive or habitual choices.

9. Satisfaction and Enjoyment: Engaging in mindful eating allows individuals to fully enjoy their food without distraction. It promotes a sense of satisfaction and pleasure from eating, as each bite is savored and appreciated.

10. **Mind-Body Connection:** Mindful eating fosters a stronger mind-body connection by promoting a deeper understanding of how food affects the body. This awareness can lead to a greater appreciation for the impact of food choices on overall health and well-being.

TIPS FOR PRACTICING MINDFUL EATING

Practicing mindful eating involves cultivating a conscious and non-judgmental awareness of your eating habits. It's about being present in the moment and fully engaging with the experience of eating. Here are some practical tips to help you incorporate mindful eating into your daily routine:

1. **Slow Down:** Take the time to slow down your eating pace. Put your utensils down between bites, chew your food thoroughly, and savor each bite. Eating slowly allows you to fully experience the flavors, textures, and aromas of your food.

2. **Remove Distractions:** Minimize distractions during meals. Turn off the TV, put away electronic devices, and focus solely on your meal. By eliminating distractions, you can give your full attention to the act of eating.

3. Engage Your Senses: Pay attention to the sensory aspects of your food. Notice the colors, smells, and textures. Take small bites and chew slowly, allowing yourself to fully experience the taste and mouthfeel of each morsel.

4. Check-In with Hunger and Fullness: Before you start eating, pause for a moment and assess your level of hunger. Similarly, throughout your meal, periodically check in with your fullness level. This helps you tune in to your body's signals and eat in accordance with your physical needs.

5. Practice Gratitude: Before you begin eating, take a moment to express gratitude for your food. Consider the effort that went into its production, the farmers and producers involved, and the nourishment it provides. Cultivating gratitude can enhance the enjoyment and appreciation of your meal.

6. Notice Emotional Triggers: Be mindful of any emotional triggers that may influence your eating habits. Notice if you're eating out of boredom, stress, or other emotions rather than true physical hunger. Pause and reflect on your emotions before reaching for food.

7. Portion Awareness: Pay attention to portion sizes and serve yourself reasonable amounts. Avoid mindlessly eating from large bags or containers. Instead, portion out your food and sit ndown at a designated eating area to promote a mindful eating environment.

8. Practice Mindful Snacking: Extend the practice of mindful eating to your snacks. Rather than mindlessly reaching for snacks, take a moment to decide if you're truly hungry or if you're eating out of habit or boredom. Choose nutrient-dense snacks and savor each bite mindfully.

9. Practice Mindful Cooking: Extend mindfulness to the cooking process as well. Engage all your senses while preparing meals, and appreciate the ingredients and techniques involved. Cooking mindfully can enhance your connection with food and the overall eating experience.

10. Be Non-Judgmental: Practice self-compassion and non-judgment during mindful eating. Let go of any guilt or negative thoughts related to food choices. Approach each eating experience with kindness and acceptance, focusing on nourishing your body and enjoying the process.

Note that, mindful eating is a practice that takes time and patience to develop. Start by incorporating these tips into a few meals or snacks each week and gradually expand from there. With consistent effort, mindful eating can become a natural part of your daily routine, allowing you to fully enjoy and appreciate your meals while nourishing your body and mind.

RECOGNIZING HUNGER AND FULLNESS CUES

Hunger and fullness cues may vary from one person to another and these can be influenced by factors such as activity levels, stress, and individual metabolism. It's important to listen to your body's signals and develop a personal understanding of your own hunger and fullness patterns. With practice, you can become more attuned to these cues, make informed choices about when and what to eat, and develop a healthier relationship with food. Recognizing hunger and fullness cues is a fundamental aspect of mindful eating. Tuning in to your body's signals and can help you establish a healthier and more balanced relationship with food. Here are some key notes on recognizing hunger and fullness cues:

1. Hunger Cues:

- Physical Sensations: Pay attention to physical sensations in your body that indicate hunger. These

may include stomach rumbling, a hollow feeling in your stomach, or a gradual decrease in energy levels.
- Thoughts and Focus: Notice if you find yourself frequently thinking about food or feeling preoccupied with thoughts of eating. This may be a sign that your body is signaling hunger.
- Time Since Last Meal: Recognize the time that has passed since your last meal or snack. As your body digests food, hunger gradually builds up.
- Gradual Increase: Hunger often builds gradually. It starts as mild discomfort and intensifies over time. Learning to recognize these subtle cues can help you respond to hunger appropriately.

2. Fullness Cues:

- Satiety Sensations: Pay attention to physical sensations of satisfaction and fullness during and after a meal. These may include a feeling of contentment, a sense of being comfortably satisfied, or a decrease in appetite.
- Slowing Down: Notice if you find yourself eating more slowly or feeling less interested in food. This may indicate that your body is signaling fullness.
- Mindful Eating Practices: Engage in mindful eating practices such as chewing food thoroughly, taking breaks between bites, and savoring the flavors. These practices can help you become more aware of the signs of fullness.

- Stomach Comfort: Check in with your stomach's physical sensations. It should feel comfortably full, but not overly stuffed or uncomfortable.

- Mind-Body Connection: Develop a strong mind-body connection by paying attention to the subtle signals your body sends during a meal. This allows you to recognize when you've had enough to eat.

3. Mindful Eating Tips for Recognizing Hunger and Fullness:

-Check-In: Pause and check in with yourself before, during, and after meals. Assess your hunger and fullness levels, and make conscious decisions about when to start and stop eating.

- Eat Mindfully: Practice mindful eating techniques such as eating slowly, savoring each bite, and engaging all your senses. This helps you stay attuned to your body's signals.

- Portion Control: Serve yourself reasonable portions and resist the urge to clean your plate if you're already feeling satisfied.

- Emotional Awareness: Distinguish between physical hunger and emotional or stress-related eating. Be aware of any emotional triggers that may influence your desire to eat.

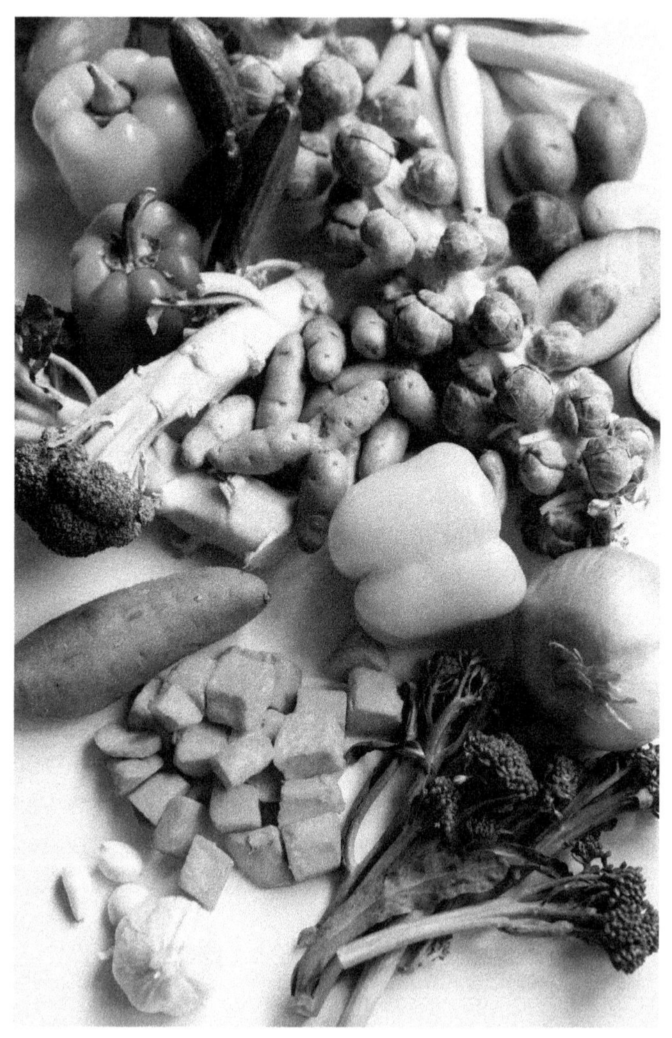

CHAPTER8: HEALTHIER CHOICES WHEN EATING AT RESTAURANTS OR ORDERING TAKEOUT

Eating out at restaurants or ordering takeout can be enjoyable and convenient, but it can also present challenges when trying to make healthy choices. However, with a mindful approach and some knowledge, you can still prioritize your health while dining out. Making healthier choices when eating out is about balance and mindful decision-making. Don't be too hard on yourself if you occasionally indulge in less healthy options. Focus on overall dietary patterns and making choices that align with your health goals. By incorporating these tips, you can enjoy dining out while still prioritizing your health. Here are some tips for making healthier choices when eating at restaurants or ordering takeout:

1. Plan Ahead:

- Research the Menu: Look up the menu online before going to the restaurant or placing your order. Identify healthier options or dishes that can be modified to fit your dietary preferences.
- Portion Sizes: Be mindful of portion sizes. Restaurant meals are often larger than what we need. Consider sharing a dish with a friend or opting for smaller portion sizes if available.

2. Choose Nutrient-Dense Options:

- Load Up on Veggies: Look for dishes that incorporate a variety of vegetables. Salads, stir-fries, or veggie-based options can be great choices for getting essential nutrients and fiber.
- Lean Protein: Opt for lean protein sources such as grilled chicken, fish, or legumes. These choices offer essential amino acids without excessive saturated fats.
- Whole Grains: Choose whole grain options like brown rice, quinoa, or whole wheat bread for added fiber and nutrients.

3. Mindful Modifications:

- Customize Your Order: Don't be afraid to ask for modifications to meet your dietary needs. Request steamed or grilled options instead of fried, ask for dressings or sauces on the side, or substitute ingredients to make the dish healthier.
- Reduce Added Sugars: Be cautious of dishes that are heavy in added sugars, such as sugary sauces or desserts. Opt for naturally sweetened options or enjoy fruit as a healthier alternative.

4. Be Mindful of Preparation Methods:

- Grilled or Baked: Choose dishes that are grilled, baked, or roasted instead of fried. This reduces the amount of unhealthy fats and calories in the meal.
- Sauce Awareness: Pay attention to the sauces and dressings used in the dishes. Many sauces can be high in sodium, sugar, or unhealthy fats. Request lighter dressings or sauces on the side, allowing you to control the amount you consume.

5. Stay Hydrated:

- Choose Water or Unsweetened Beverages: Opt for water, unsweetened tea, or sparkling water instead of sugary beverages. This helps reduce unnecessary added sugars and keeps you hydrated.

6. Practice Portion Control:

- Share or Save: Consider sharing a dish with a friend or family member. If that's not possible, ask for a to-go box in advance and save a portion of the meal for later. This prevents overeating and allows you to enjoy the meal over multiple sittings.

7. Enjoy Mindfully:

- Slow Down and Savor: Take your time to eat and enjoy the flavors and textures of your food. Eating slowly helps you recognize when you're full and prevents overeating.
- Practice Moderation: While it's important to make healthier choices, it's also okay to indulge occasionally. Balance your meal with healthier

options and allow yourself to enjoy a treat in moderation.

NAVIGATING MENUS AND PORTION SIZES

By being aware of your choices and portion sizes, you can make healthier decisions while still enjoying dining out.When it comes to navigating menus and managing portion sizes, here are a few strategies you can consider:

1.Plan ahead: Before you go to a restaurant or order food, take a moment to review the menu online if available. Look for healthier options or dishes that align with your dietary goals. Having a plan can help you make better choices when faced with numerous options.

2.Watch for keywords: Pay attention to descriptive words used in menu items. Words like "grilled," "steamed," or "baked" generally indicate healthier preparation methods. On the other hand, terms like "fried," "crispy," or "creamy" often suggest higher calorie content.

3.Portion control: Many restaurants serve larger portions than what is recommended for a single meal. Consider sharing an entrée with a friend or opting for a smaller-sized portion if available. You can also ask for a to-go box at the beginning of the meal and pack away half of your meal before you start eating.

4.Balance your plate: Aim for a well-balanced meal that includes protein, vegetables, whole grains, and healthy fats. Look for options that offer a variety of food groups and avoid dishes that are predominantly high in one category, such as fried foods or heavy pasta dishes.

5.Be mindful of extras: Pay attention to extras like dressings, sauces, and condiments, as they can add extra calories and sodium to your meal. Ask for dressings and sauces on the side, so you can control the amount you use or opt for healthier alternatives like lemon juice or vinegar.

6.Drink wisely: Be mindful of calorie-laden beverages such as sugary sodas, cocktails, or creamy coffee drinks. Choose water, unsweetened tea, or other low-calorie options to accompany your meal.

TIPS FOR ENJOYING SOCIAL MEALS

The goal is to find a balance between enjoying social meals and maintaining healthy habits as long as you practice moderation and make conscious choices. Here are some tips to help you enjoy social meals while maintaining healthy habits:

1.Communicate your preferences:

Let your friends or family know about your commitment to healthy eating. By communicating your preferences, they can be more considerate when planning meals or choosing restaurants. You may even find that others in your social circle have similar goals and can support each other.

2.Plan ahead: If you know you have a social meal coming up, plan your other meals and snacks accordingly. Make healthier choices leading up to the event to create a calorie buffer, allowing you to indulge a bit more during the social meal.

3.Be selective: When faced with a buffet or a wide variety of food options, take a lap around the table before making your choices. Assess the available options and select the foods that align with your health goals. Focus on lean proteins, vegetables, whole grains, and fruits, and be mindful of portion sizes.

4.Mindful eating: Practice mindful eating techniques during social meals. Slow down, savor each bite, and pay attention to your body's hunger and fullness cues. By eating more slowly and being

present in the moment, you can enjoy your meal and prevent overeating.

5.Control portions: If the portions served are larger than what you need, consider splitting an entrée with a friend or asking for a to-go box right at the beginning of the meal to pack away any excess food. This way, you can enjoy the meal without feeling obligated to finish everything on your plate.

6.Hydrate wisely: Be mindful of your beverage choices during social meals. Opt for water, unsweetened beverages, or light options instead of sugary drinks or alcoholic beverages, which can contribute excess calories.

7.Be active together: Plan social activities that involve physical movement, such as going for a walk or playing a sport. This can help balance out any indulgences during the meal and keep you engaged in a healthy lifestyle.

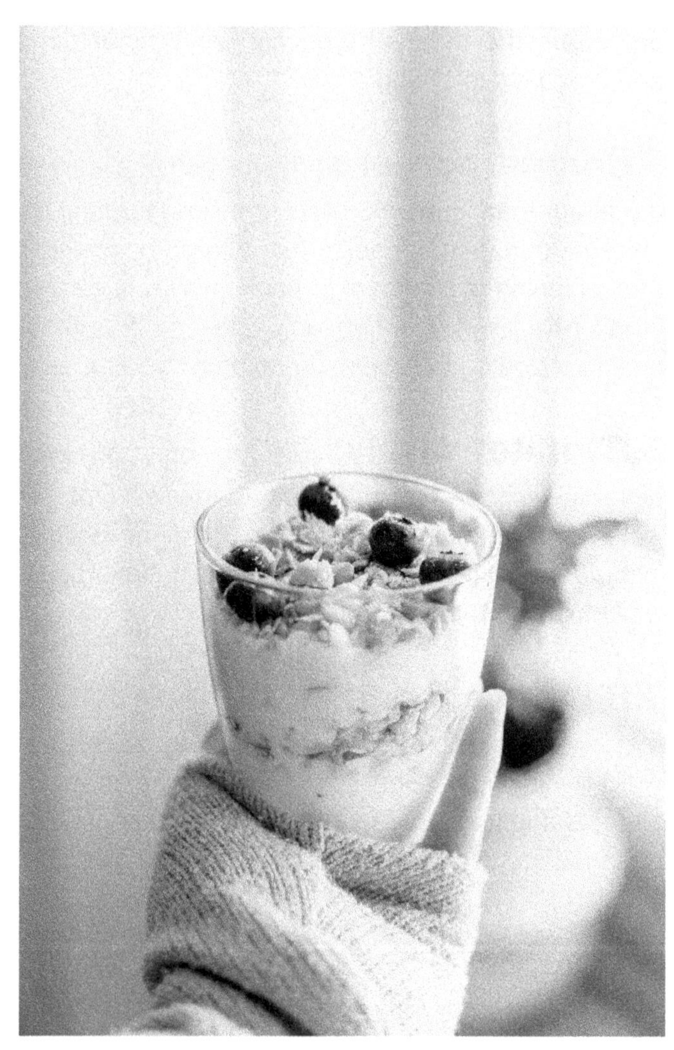

CHAPTER 9: IMPORTANCE OF BALANCE AND FLEXIBILITY IN A HEALTHY EATING PLAN

Balance and flexibility work hand in hand to create a sustainable and enjoyable approach to healthy eating. They help prevent feelings of deprivation, promote long-term adherence to a healthy lifestyle, and support mental and emotional well-being in relation to food.

Balanced eating also means avoiding excessive consumption of any particular food or nutrient while focusing on moderation and portion control. It emphasizes the importance of including a diverse array of foods to promote overall well-being and prevent nutrient deficiencies. Balance involves incorporating a variety of foods from different food groups in appropriate proportions to meet your nutritional needs. A balanced eating plan typically includes a combination of fruits, vegetables, whole grains, lean proteins, and healthy fats. It ensures that you receive a wide range of essential nutrients, such as vitamins, minerals, proteins, carbohydrates, and fats, for optimal health.

Flexibility in a healthy eating plan allows for individual preferences, dietary needs, and various situations. It acknowledges that everyone has unique tastes, cultural considerations, ethical choices, and health restrictions. Flexibility means being adaptable and making choices that align with your personal circumstances while still promoting overall health.

Flexibility also encompasses the ability to accommodate social gatherings, special occasions, and eating out. It means being able to enjoy meals without rigidly sticking to a specific meal plan. It involves making informed choices, being mindful of portion sizes, and finding a balance between nourishing your body and indulging in occasional treats.

Balance and flexibility are crucial components of a healthy eating plan. Here's why they are important:

1.Nutritional adequacy: A balanced

eating plan ensures that you receive a wide range of nutrients necessary for good health. By including foods from different food groups in appropriate proportions, you can meet your body's nutrient requirements, including vitamins, minerals, proteins, carbohydrates, and healthy fats.

2.Variety and enjoyment:

Eating a diverse range of foods not only helps prevent nutrient deficiencies but also adds excitement and enjoyment to your meals. Incorporating various flavors, textures, and colors makes eating more pleasurable and can help prevent food monotony, which can lead to boredom or cravings.

3.Sustainable lifestyle:

A balanced and flexible approach to eating is more sustainable in the long term. It allows you to include a wide variety of foods, including occasional treats, without feeling deprived or restricted. This makes it easier to stick to your healthy eating plan over time, promoting consistency and preventing feelings of frustration or guilt.

4.Individual preferences and needs:

Each person has unique preferences, dietary needs, and cultural or ethical considerations. A flexible eating plan allows for customization based on these factors. It accommodates personal food choices, restrictions, or allergies, making it easier to adhere to a healthy lifestyle that suits your individual circumstances.

5.Social situations and flexibility:

Social gatherings, special occasions, and eating out are part of our lives. Flexibility in your eating plan allows you to navigate these situations without feeling stressed or excluded. It enables you to make thoughtful choices, enjoy special meals, and maintain a healthy balance overall.

6.Mental and emotional well-being:

An overly rigid eating plan can lead to feelings of deprivation, guilt, or anxiety around food. By embracing balance and flexibility, you develop a healthier relationship with food. It promotes a positive mindset, reduces stress associated with strict dietary rules, and fosters a more relaxed approach to eating.

Balance and flexibility do not mean disregarding your health goals entirely. They involve making mindful choices, being aware of portion sizes, and finding the right equilibrium that supports your overall well-being while allowing for occasional indulgences.

REALISTIC EXPECTATIONS AND GRADUAL LIFESTYLE CHANGES

Encouraging realistic expectations and gradual lifestyle changes is crucial for sustainable and long-term success. It's important to understand that significant changes don't happen overnight and that setting achievable goals is key to staying motivated. By adopting a gradual approach, individuals can create a positive environment for personal growth and development.

Realistic expectations help prevent disappointment and frustration. Instead of aiming for drastic transformations, focus on setting small, attainable goals that contribute to a larger vision. Breaking down big goals into smaller milestones allows for a sense of accomplishment along the way. This approach keeps motivation high and builds momentum for further progress.

Lifestyle changes should be approached gradually to ensure they become lasting habits. Rather than attempting an abrupt overhaul, identify one or two areas you'd like to improve and work on them systematically. For example, if you want to adopt a healthier lifestyle, start by incorporating small changes like adding more fruits and vegetables to your diet or increasing physical activity gradually. As these changes become routine, you can build upon them and take further steps toward your desired lifestyle.

It's important to remember that sustainable change takes time and consistency. Be patient with yourself and celebrate every small victory along the way. Embrace the journey of self-improvement, and don't be discouraged by setbacks. Remember that setbacks are opportunities to learn and adjust your approach. By maintaining realistic expectations and embracing gradual lifestyle changes, you'll increase your chances of long-term success and a more fulfilling life.

HOW TO ADDRESS COMMON CHALLENGES AND STRATEGIES FOR OVERCOMING THEM

To address common challenges and offering strategies for overcoming them is essential for personal growth and success. By acknowledging and tackling these challenges head-on, you can develop effective strategies to overcome obstacles and achieve your goals. Here are some general steps to address common challenges:

1.Identify the Challenge: Start by recognizing the specific challenge you're facing. Whether it's related to time management, motivation, or a particular skill, understanding the nature of the challenge is crucial.

2.Analyze the Root Cause: Dig deeper to identify the underlying causes of the challenge. Is it a lack of knowledge, external factors, or internal barriers? Pinpointing the root cause helps you address it more effectively.

3.Seek Support and Guidance: Reach out to others who have faced similar challenges or seek professional assistance. This could involve talking to a mentor, joining support groups, or consulting experts in the field. They can provide valuable insights, advice, and strategies based on their experiences.

4.Set Realistic Goals: Establish clear, specific, and attainable goals related to overcoming the challenge. Break them down into smaller milestones, making it easier to track progress and maintain motivation.

5.Develop Strategies and Action Plans: Create a plan of action tailored to the challenge at hand. Determine the steps you need to take, and consider potential obstacles and alternative approaches. Having a well-defined strategy enhances your chances of success.

6.Build Habits and Consistency: Consistency is key to addressing challenges. Incorporate new habits and practices into your daily routine that support your goals. Gradually integrate these changes, making them more sustainable and manageable.

7.Stay Motivated and Positive: Maintaining a positive mindset and finding motivation along the way Is cruclal. Celebrate small victories, practice self-care, and surround yourself with positive influences. Remember that setbacks are opportunities for growth, and focus on the progress you've made.

8.Review and Adjust: Regularly assess your progress and adjust your strategies as needed. Be flexible and open to refining your approach based on what works best for you. Continual evaluation and adaptation increase your chances of overcoming challenges effectively.

But remember, each individual's journey is unique, and what works for one person may not work for another. Be patient with yourself, practice self-compassion, and approach challenges as opportunities for personal growth. With determination, perseverance, and the right strategies, you can overcome common challenges and achieve your desired outcomes.

CHAPTER 10: RECAPS OF THE KEY POINTS DISCUSSED

By incorporating the following key points into your approach, you'll be better equipped to develop and maintain healthy eating habits. Stay committed, be patient with yourself, and enjoy the journey of improving your overall health and well-being. Here's a recap of the key points discussed throughout the guide on healthy eating habits:

1.Realistic Expectations and Gradual Changes: Set achievable goals and embrace a gradual approach to sustainable and long-term success.

2.Common Challenges and Strategies:

•

A.Temptation and Cravings: Keep unhealthy foods out of sight, practice mindful eating, and find healthier alternatives.

B.Busy Lifestyle: Plan and prepare meals in advance, opt for quick and easy recipes, and pack healthy snacks.

C.Emotional Eating: Identify triggers, find alternative ways to manage emotions, and practice self-care activities.

D.Lack of Knowledge: Educate yourself about balanced nutrition, experiment with new recipes, and consult a registered dietitian.

E.Social Pressures: Communicate your health goals, bring healthy dishes to social events, and focus on socializing rather than solely on food.

3.Addressing Challenges:

A.Identify the challenge and analyze the root cause.

B.Seek support and guidance from mentors, support groups, or experts.

C.Set realistic goals and develop strategies and action plans.

D.Build habits and consistency by integrating changes into your routine.
Stay motivated, positive, and celebrate small victories.

E.Regularly review and adjust your strategies based on progress and needs.

4.Personalization and Flexibility:

Remember that everyone's journey is unique, so tailor the strategies to your own preferences and needs. Be flexible and open to adjustments along the way.

HOW TO START INCORPORATING HEALTHY EATING HABITS INTO YOUR DAILY LIFE

For you to start incorporating healthy eating habits into your daily life, remember that every positive change begins with a single decision, and your commitment to a healthier lifestyle is truly commendable.Starting may feel overwhelming, but keep in mind that small steps can lead to significant transformations. Begin by focusing on one aspect of your diet that you'd like to improve. It could be adding more fruits and vegetables, reducing processed foods, or drinking more water. Choose an area that resonates with you and aligns with your goals.To make the transition easier, try incorporating healthy choices gradually. Start by replacing one unhealthy snack with a nutritious alternative or swapping a sugary drink with water or herbal tea. Celebrate these small victories as they bring you closer to your ultimate goal.

Additionally, make meal planning and preparation a priority. Dedicate some time each week to plan your meals, create a grocery list, and batch cook or pre-cut ingredients for convenience. This way, you'll have healthier options readily available when hunger strikes or when you're pressed for time.

Remember, healthy eating isn't about deprivation or strict diets. It's about nourishing your body with wholesome, nutrient-rich foods that make you feel energized and vibrant. Embrace a balanced approach, including a variety of food groups, and savor each meal mindfully, paying attention to your body's hunger and fullness cues.Surround yourself with support and encouragement. Share your goals with loved ones and seek their support on your journey. Consider joining online communities or seeking guidance from professionals who can provide insights, motivation, and helpful tips.
Most importantly, be kind to yourself. Acknowledge that change takes time and setbacks are a natural part of the process. If you have an off day or indulge in something less nutritious, don't let it discourage you. Instead, use it as an opportunity to learn and reaffirm your commitment to making healthier choices moving forward.You're capable of making positive changes, and by incorporating healthy eating habits into your daily life, you're investing in your well-being and long-term happiness. Believe in yourself, stay motivated, and enjoy the rewarding journey of nourishing your body and embracing a healthier lifestyle.

ADDITIONAL RESOURCES AND REFERENCES:

Here are some additional resources and references for further exploration on healthy eating habits:

1.   Websites and Online Resources:
•   Mayo Clinic Nutrition and Healthy Eating (https://www.mayoclinic.org/healthy-lifestyle/nutrition-and-healthy-eating)
•   National Institute of Diabetes and Digestive and Kidney Diseases (NIDDK) - Healthy Eating and Nutrition (https://www.niddk.nih.gov/health-information/weight-management/healthy-eating-nutrition)
•   American Heart Association - Healthy Eating (https://www.heart.org/en/healthy-living/healthy-eating)
•   Academy of Nutrition and Dietetics (https://www.eatright.org/)
2.   Books:
•   "In Defense of Food: An Eater's Manifesto" by Michael Pollan
•   "The Blue Zones Kitchen: 100 Recipes to Live to 100" by Dan Buettner
•   "Food Rules: An Eater's Manual" by Michael Pollan
•   "How Not to Die: Discover the Foods Scientifically Proven to Prevent and Reverse Disease" by Michael Greger

3.	Mobile Apps:
•	MyFitnessPal: A popular app for tracking calories, macronutrients, and exercise.
•	Fooducate: Helps you make healthier food choices by providing nutrition information and product recommendations.
•	HealthyOut: Allows you to find healthy restaurant meals near you based on your dietary preferences.
4.	Registered Dietitians and Nutritionists:
•	Consulting a registered dietitian or nutritionist can provide personalized guidance and support based on your specific needs and goals.

These resources offer a wealth of information, expert advice, recipes, and tools to help you delve deeper into healthy eating habits and nutrition. Remember to always evaluate and verify the information you come across, ensuring it aligns with reputable sources and scientific evidence.

Enjoy your exploration, and may these resources empower you on your journey to a healthier lifestyle!

www.ingramcontent.com/pod-product-compliance
Lightning Source LLC
Chambersburg PA
CBHW071607270726
48661CB00019B/1619